Yoga

20 Essential Yoga Poses for Improving Your Health, Reducing Stress & Anxiety, Increasing Your Energy, and Losing Weight!

Catherine Walker

Catherine Walker

Table Of Contents

Introduction

I want to thank you and congratulate you for downloading the book, "Yoga: 20 Essential Yoga Poses for Improving Your Health, Reducing Stress & Anxiety, Increasing Your Energy, and Losing Weight!".

This book contains proven steps and strategies on how to make use of different yoga poses to achieve the healthier, slimmer, more energetic, and stress-free body you have long desired.

More than just a simple fitness routine to add to your arsenal of long-given-up-on workout fads, yoga is a unique combination of breath control, meditation, fitness training, and gymnastics. This book aims to help you learn the proper way of performing different poses so that you can live a healthy and fit life that is full of energy and free from stress.

Thanks again for downloading this book. I truly hope you enjoy it and benefit from all that it has to offer!

Chapter 1: Getting Acquainted: Yoga Essentials To Learn

The Yoga Method

The yoga lifestyle is one that involves both the mind and the body. Practiced for more than five thousand years, yoga can hardly be considered as a mere workout fad.

The reason for yoga's long-standing popularity could be because it is a form of exercise that does not only help you burn fat as well as work your muscles, but also because it allows you to feel relaxed and energized at the same time. Yoga is an overall mind-body workout, combining a number of stretching and strengthening poses with relaxation, meditation, and deep breathing. For best results and comfort, yoga should be practiced on an empty stomach.

Gains To Be Had

Yoga benefits you in a number of ways:

Yoga is a low-impact way of *improving your health*. With yoga, you can rest assured that your body gets a full workout without your joints being strained.

Yoga is as good as any type of aerobic exercise in helping you *lose weight*. The more athletic forms of yoga allow you to work up a good sweat, burn off calories, and shed excess weight.

Practicing yoga, especially on a regular basis, helps a lot in *reducing your stress* as you are allowed to stretch your muscles as well as increase your range of motion.

Increasing your energy levels is possible with the aid of various yoga poses, which effectively strengthen different muscles in your body as you hold them in balanced positions.

Different Strokes For Different Folks

There are many forms of yoga you can try, including the following:

Ashtanga refers to poses performed in a series that let you make use of special breathing techniques.

Bikram or "hot yoga" involves a number of challenging poses that require you to work out in an area that is heated to high temperatures.

Hatha is a mix of basic yoga movements and breathing.

Iyengar helps you properly align your body with the use of straps, blocks, and chairs.

Power yoga refers to a form of yoga that lets you build your muscles with its faster and higher-intensity method.

Vinyasa involves performing different poses one after the other in a smooth-flowing manner.

Yin Yoga refers to a form of yoga where poses are held longer than usual (up to 5 minutes in length) in order to stretch connective tissue.

Target Sighted

Different areas of your body are targeted by yoga:

Arms. Yoga lets you build up your arm strength without having to use machines or weights; instead, it encourages you to use your own body weight.

Back. Your back muscles get a good stretch from performing yoga, which is the reason yoga is effective in providing relief for a sore back.

Core. Every core muscle in your body gets a good workout when you perform yoga poses. For example, you may prop your body up on a single arm or keep your legs upright in the air as you balance your body on your sitting bones if your goal is to tighten your flabby stomach.

Glutes. Sculpt your backside with a number of yoga poses.

Legs. Your thighs, hips, quadriceps, hamstrings, and calves get a good workout from yoga.

Chapter 2: High Five: 5 Yoga Poses For Improved Health

Having a healthier body does not necessarily mean running laps until your sneaker's soles are worn out or sweating it out at the gym until you collapse. Here are five not-so-easy but definitely doable yoga poses you can perform right in the comfort of your own home.

General tips:

Know that breathing plays an important role in yoga. It will help a lot in preventing any feelings of discomfort while you are holding a particular pose for an extended period of time. Plus, filling your body with fresh air also lets you breathe out "negative vibes".

Make sure to take deep and slow breaths throughout each yoga pose you perform. Try to breathe in and out through your nose.

Try staying in each yoga pose for 5 to 7 full breaths; it is much easier to measure how long you should stay in each pose by counting number of breaths, as opposed to length of time.

Before you repeat a pose on your other side, it is best to release said pose on the first side after you exhale.

Yoga poses for improving your health:

SUPPORTED HEADSTAND POSE

Benefits:

Strengthening of your deep core muscles

Flushing of your blood as well as the oxygen and nutrients it carries to your brain glands (pituitary and hypothalamus)

Improving digestion as well as circulation

Improving depression and concentration

Steps:

1. Position yourself on your knees and hands. Making sure that both your elbows are aligned under your shoulders, put your forearms on the yoga mat.

2. As you bring your left and right hands together, allow the top of your head to lower to the mat. Place your head on the cup made by your interlaced fingers.

3. Pressing your two wrists into the mat, gently press the back of your head with your thumbs.

4. Let your toes curl under, and then breathe in as you walk your feet in the direction of your elbows. See to it that you press your forearms down, wrist to elbow – this will help firm your shoulder blades against your back. Doing so also ensures that your shoulders are prevented from collapsing and that you do not place too much weight on both your head and neck.

Remember:

When lifting both your legs into a headstand, raise your left leg up first. You can then simply bring the right leg up to meet the left one.

If you are having a bit of trouble performing this pose, it helps to make sure to draw back your lower ribs, tuck your tailbone up in the direction of the ceiling, engage the muscles in your thighs, and reach up into the balls of your feet through your legs.

Make sure to align the center arches of your two feet with the middle part of your pelvis (this area aligns above the crown of your head).

As you come out of this yoga position, ensure that you keep pressing with the help of your forearms.

Practicing this yoga pose in front of your living room or bedroom wall can help reduce your nervousness about doing a headstand for the first time.

You may not like the idea of having one foot up and then having the other foot meet it. What you can do instead is to raise your two feet at the same time: Bend your knees into your chest, then gradually raise your knees in the direction of the ceiling before you finally straighten your two legs.

You have to be extra careful in doing this yoga pose if you have a heart condition, eye infection, are menstruating, are prone to severe headaches, are suffering from a neck or back injury, or have high blood pressure that is uncontrollable.

DISCLAIMER - It is strongly recommended that you perform this yoga pose the first few times under the guidance of a trained yoga professional.

FISH TWIST POSE

Benefits:

Relief of symptoms of backache

Stimulation of digestion

Provide boost to your kidneys and liver

Strengthening of your spine

Provide flexibility to your neck, shoulder, and hips

Great stimulation for thyroid gland

Steps:

1. Sit down on the yoga mat and then bring your two legs forward. With your legs straightened, bend your left knee towards your chest area while crossing your left foot over your right thigh.

2. Making sure that your left knee is up and your left foot is flat on the mat, shift the weight of your body to your right hip, bending your right knee so that your right heel comes to your left hip in an outward direction.

3. Allow your weight to be distributed onto your left and right hip areas comfortably. Put your left hand on the mat behind your left hip and sit tall. Press sitting bones down and lift your torso up as you breathe in. As you breathe out, gently twist to the left while keeping your sitting bones down.

4. Maintain for 5-7 breaths.

Remember:

You will be able to perform this yoga pose with a deeper twist by bringing your right arm to the outer part of your left knee. Make sure to keep your elbows bent.

In twisting your body from the core of your torso, let your abs do the work; see to it that your front torso and inner left thigh are pulled together. Gaze over your shoulder (left or right) by swiveling your head.

When breathing in, make sure that you lift your chest high and that your spine is lengthened.

It helps to twist your torso a bit deeper with each exhalation.

You can elevate your hips by sitting on a blanket that has been folded. This is particularly helpful if you feel unbalanced, have tight hamstrings, or if this pose adds discomfort to your lower back.

If it is too much, you can straighten your bottom leg and point your toes up to the ceiling.

Breathe out as you get into the twist and reach for the wall at your back. Make sure that your arm is almost, but not quite, fully extended.

To allow your torso to get closer to your thigh, keep on reaching for the wall.

HALF-MOON ON THE BALANCE POSE

Benefits:

Strengthening and toning of your muscles

Increase of body awareness and balance

Relief of stress

Improves balance

Steps:

1. Stand with your two feet placed together on the yoga mat. Hinge your body forward at the hip area and then press your palms down into the mat. See to it that your chest remains even, above, or with your hips. You can use a block, stool, or chair if your palms don't reach the floor. It is key that you perform this exercise with straight legs.

2. Engage your abdominal muscles as you squeeze the blades of your shoulders together. This will help to ensure that you will be performing this pose with a tabletop-flat back.

3. Control your body as you lift your right leg and keep the hip height at your back. Make sure that your ankles are kept flexed and that your toes are pulled back in the direction of your face.

4. To help you maintain your balance while performing this yoga pose, engage your abdominal muscles as well as your entire right leg.

Remember:

At your own pace, place your right palm on your right hip. You may have to move your left hand to the left side about ten inches away from your left pinky toe's front.

It helps to fix your gaze at the yoga mat as you gradually bring your right hip on top of your left hip. This opens your body to the wall at your side.

As you get comfortable, lift your arm towards the ceiling and point your fingertips up. Make sure to stack your wrist directly on top of your shoulder.

Try reaching through your right fingertips as you keep pressing your left palm into the mat.

If you find it difficult to start doing this yoga pose with a flat back as well as keeping your chest aligned with your hips, you may use something stable (like a block) to keep your body leveled out and offer added balancing support at the same time.

BRIDGE POSE

Benefits:

Provide flexibility to your spine, neck, shoulders, chest, and hips

Offer calmness to your nervous system

Reduction of stress, insomnia, anxiety, and depression

Improvement of digestion

Steps:

1. Lie on your back on the yoga mat. With both your arms placed at your sides, bend your left and right knees and keep soles of your feet flat on the mat. Make sure your feet are close to the bones that you sit on so that your fingertips may touch your heels.

2. See to it that your feet and thighs are in line and parallel with your hips.

3. Press your feet into the mat as you raise your pelvic, lower back, and upper back areas prior to interlacing the fingers of your hands under your tailbone. Some people may not be able to interlace their fingers under their tailbone due to tight shoulders. Only perform this maneuver in full if you feel comfortable with it. Don't force movements that put further strain on your body.

4. Press both your left and right arms into the mat as you raise your chest towards your chin. Make sure that you roll underneath the outer sides of your arms.

Remember:

See to it that the only parts of your body touching the ground are your head (back portion), outer arms, and feet.

Engage the top portions of your thighs in this yoga pose by pressing your heels down towards your front without having to move your feet.

When performing the bridge pose, make sure that your hamstrings and glutes are relaxed and that your inner thighs are spun down in the direction of the mat.

If your shoulders' back portions are bothered, you will find that placing a folded towel or blanket beneath them helps.

Note: Never turn your head to the side when in Bridge Pose.

Do away with this pose if you are suffering from a neck injury.

SIDE-TWISTING SHOULDER STAND POSE

Benefits:

Improve blood circulation

Flushing of the lymphatic systems in your underarm, abdomen, and groin areas

Better digestion

Steps:

1. Lie down on the yoga mat. Protect your neck from pressure by inserting three folded blankets between your shoulders and the yoga mat so that there is a small area of space in between your neck and the blankets and so that your head is on the floor (not on the blankets).

2. Start by stabilizing your elbows and the back of your arms on the floor. Place your hands on either side of your lower back. Then, lift only your torso and bend your knees. Afterwards, slowly raise your legs up vertically.

3. Accomplish a shoulder stand by lengthening your torso in the direction of the ceiling until your hands find their way onto your rib cage. Climb your hands as high as possible up your back while keeping your elbows in.

4. Note: This is a difficult pose. Allow your legs to lower towards your face if you feel that the vertical extension of your legs is too difficult to maintain. This adjustment should take a lot of pressure off of the shoulder girdle.

Remember:

Twist your abdomen and hips in a single direction. I recommend doing this with a trained yoga instructor as it is a difficult pose. I only advise doing the twisting movement if you are in a perfectly aligned shoulder stand, with your legs straight up and strong. Your shoulders and head must be completely stable.

Make sure that your neck is not strained as you perform this pose so that your shoulders are not distorted.

Keep your legs in place by using your abdominal muscles. Then do a backbend by extending your spine and lengthening your navel.

Note: Never turn your head to the side when doing a Shoulder Stand.

Chapter 3 : Lighten Up: 5 Stress-Reducing Yoga Poses

The first step to reducing your stress with the aid of yoga is to move past certain preconceptions, one of which being that you need to have a flexible body in order to perform yoga. The truth is that individuals who do not have much flexibility in their body are actually going to see results more quickly. It is also important to note that a yoga beginner (like you may be) should not worry about executing every yoga pose *perfectly*. And please know that there is absolutely no need to memorize the names of these yoga poses – it may only stress you out more. Just try to get the movements down to the best of your ability. Keep trying until you get them right, because a guide like this is essentially useless unless you apply what you are learning!

General tips:

Focusing on your breath is essential in doing yoga to reduce your stress. When you concentrate on how you are breathing in and out, you are allowing yourself to savor the present moment, let go of any worries, and eliminate stress.

Know that doing yoga is not about being better or worse at it than anybody else. No two individuals perform a yoga pose in the exact the same way. Strive to do the poses at your own pace and level of flexibility. The key is to feel challenged, not overwhelmed.

Yoga poses for reducing stress:

MOUNTAIN POSE

Benefits:

Besides providing stress relief, doing the mountain pose in the right way can help a lot in improving your balance and posture.

Steps:

1. Stand with your heels very slightly apart (big toes lightly touching), and with your arms hanging by your sides.

2. Focus your thoughts on imagining that your ankles and inner feet are lifting.

3. Stretch out your collarbones as you pull down your shoulder blades.

4. Align your head with your shoulders while making sure that your chin is parallel to the yoga mat.

5. Hold this pose for thirty seconds to one minute.

Remember:

It is important to avoid pulling your head back or pushing it forward when doing this pose.

Avoid tucking or arching your lower back as well as pelvis.

DOG-DOWN POSE

Benefits:

Aside from reducing your stress, the dog-down pose effectively works your upper body. It also allows you to flex your back, chest, arm, and leg muscles.

Steps:

1. Position your body on all fours. Make sure your toes are turned under, your knees are below your hips, and your hands are slightly in front of your shoulders.

2. Breathe out and begin straightening your legs, seeing to it that your heels are popping up from the yoga mat.

3. Raise your sitting bones to the ceiling while pushing your heels towards the mat.

4. As you gently press your palms down into the mat, gradually straighten your arms while sliding your shoulder blades down your back.

5. Hold this position for one to three minutes.

Remember:

Keep your head relaxed.

Keep your head between your upper left and right arms.

To make sure you are breathing long and full breaths both in and out.

PLANK POSE

Benefits:

The plank pose helps you achieve stronger core muscles, wrists, and arms, as well as helping to get rid of your stress.

Perform this pose from the dog-down pose.

Steps:

1. Lower your torso in front of you, keeping your arms straight. Make sure your arms are perpendicular to the yoga mat and that your palms are situated directly below your shoulders.

2. Feel your collarbones expand as you pull the blades of your shoulders down, looking down directly at the mat.

Remember:

It is best to hold the plank pose for thirty seconds to one minute.

UPWARD DOG POSE

Benefits:

The uppity dog pose does not only condition your upper body, but it also helps to relieve you from stress.

Steps:

1. Lie down on your stomach on the yoga mat. Keep your legs straight and your feet on the mat.

2. Bend your arms at the elbows while placing your palms on the mat right beside your waist.

3. Lift your torso and the thighs off the floor by pressing your hands and tops of your feet into the mat. Remember to keep your chin tucked in.

4. Allow your shoulder blades to drop down your back. Raise your chest gently towards the ceiling. (Make sure you do this step without straining your neck area).

5. Hold this pose for fifteen seconds to a half minute.

Remember:

To tighten your abdominal muscles and pull in your belly button towards your spine.

To make sure you are breathing long and full breaths both in and out.

BUTTERFLY POSE

Benefits:

The butterfly pose allows you to reduce stress while increasing the flexibility in your hips, inner thighs, and lower back.

Steps:

1. Sit down on the yoga mat, keeping your straightened legs out in front of you.

2. Bend at the knees. Pull your heels in the direction of your groin and press the soles of your feet together.

3. Open out your bended knees to the sides.

4. Allow your two hands to reach forward until they hold onto your shins, ankles, or feet.

5. Hold this position for one to two minutes.

Remember:

Your knees can drop down closer to the mat if you relax your thighs.

To make sure you are breathing long and full breaths both in and out.

Chapter 4: Shed It Off: 5 Yoga Poses To Help You Lose Weight

When practiced with the right form and on a regular basis, yoga can help you lose excess weight, especially when you are working with a trained instructor. Yoga effectively works out your body while being light on your joints. This ensures that any chances of you getting injured are kept at a minimum. And know that the best part about doing yoga to lose weight is that you can do it right at home – no need to sign up for a costly gym membership!

General tips:

Wear comfortable clothes, lay out the yoga mat, and you are set to go.

Certain key moves are included in nearly all types of yoga poses. It would be best for you to work with an instructor to get a better visual representation of these yoga poses.

Yoga poses for weight loss:

WARRIOR ONE POSE

Benefits:

The warrior pose lets you effectively stretch your back, strengthen your tummy, thighs, and buttocks, and shed excess weight.

Steps:

1. With your left and right hands by your sides, stand while keeping your feet together.

2. Extend your left leg in front of you and your right leg behind you.

3. Gently bend your left knee as you approach the lunge position.

4. Twist your body at the torso in order to face your bended left leg.

5. Turn your right foot a bit sideways so that you gain additional support.

6. Breathe out, straighten out your arms, and lift your body away from your bended left knee and up towards the ceiling.

7. Allow your arms to stretch upwards, and then gradually tilt your torso behind you so that your back takes the form of an arch.

8. Repeat the steps with your other leg.

Remember:

Getting out of this pose is easy. Breathe out, straighten your left knee, push off your left leg, and go back to the original position.

To avoid injuring your legs or back, never rush to get out of the warrior pose.

It is best to avoid doing the warrior pose if you a have back, shoulder, or knee injury.

CHAIR POSE

Benefits:

The chair pose has the ability to strengthen not only your core muscles but your thighs and buttocks as well.

Steps:

1. With both of your hands forward, stand straight on the yoga mat.

2. Lift your hands over your head. Bend your knees so that your thighs are in a position that is parallel to the mat.

3. Breathe in as you bend slightly forward at the torso.

4. Hold this pose as long as possible before gently going back to your original position.

Remember:

Do not attempt this pose if you have an injured knee or back.

Leveled breathing will sustain you through the pose.

TUMMY WORKOUT POSE

Benefits:

The tummy workout pose is actually a type of breathing exercise that helps to improve your digestion. It also helps to bring oxygen into your body as it strengthens your stomach as well as your abdominal muscles. This kind of breathing is called Kapalabati.

Doing this pose regularly helps you achieve a flat, toned stomach.

Steps:

1. Sit down in a cross-legged fashion on the yoga mat with your palms holding onto your knees and your spine erect.

2. Breathe out through your nose. Pull in your stomach towards your spine.

3. Allow yourself to automatically breathe in as you loosen the muscles in your stomach.

4. Contract the muscles in your stomach quickly before exhaling.

5. Do 25 repetitions of this pose in the beginning. As you become more comfortable with it, you may then do more reps.

Remember:

Let your stomach muscles do all the work with regards to pushing out as well as pulling in air.

It is normal to feel a bit sore around your stomach and abdomen muscles after doing this pose.

It is best to do away with this pose if you have heart disease, a hernia, or high blood pressure.

BUTTERFLY POSE IN MOTION

Benefits:

This pose helps improves digestion as well as reduce the amount of fat located around your inner thigh area.

It also helps in the strengthening of your spine as well as lower back, knees, and groin muscles.

This pose also effectively relieves the discomfort brought about by menstruation.

Steps:

1. With your legs stretched out forward, sit comfortably on the yoga mat.

2. Bend your knees while keeping your spine erect. This will allow the soles of your feet to face each other.

3. Use your hand to pull in your legs. This allows your heels to touch one another and get close to your pelvic area.

4. Hold your left and right legs at the ankle area. Similar to a butterfly's wings, move your thighs in an up-down manner.

5. Do as many repetitions of this pose as you can.

Remember:

You will reap more benefits from the pose if you keep your legs as close to your pelvis as possible.

Avoid pushing yourself when performing this pose, especially if your knees are injured.

PLOW POSE

Benefits:

The plough pose can greatly benefit individuals who have to sit for long periods of time.

The benefits of this pose include improving bad posture, toning your buttock muscles, straightening your thighs and shoulders, stimulation of your thyroid and parathyroid glands, abdominal organs, and lungs, improvement of your digestion, and stabilizing hormone levels.

Steps:

1. Lie down on the yoga mat, keeping your back flat.

2. While placing your left and right arms by your sides, bend at the knees to keep the soles of your feet flat on the mat.

3. Gradually lift your legs at the hip area. Use your hands to support your hips as you lift them.

4. Bend your legs slowly at the hips. Allow your toes to touch the mat behind your head. Keep your hands straightened so that your palms are flat on the mat. It may be helpful to have a stool or a chair behind your head for your feet to land on; this is especially useful if you have tight hamstrings.

5. Go up while breathing out.

6. Go back to the original lying position by gently rolling your back on the mat. Breathe in as you gradually drop down.

Remember:

Avoid the plough pose if you have issues with hypertension, diarrhea, a neck injury, spleen or liver disorders, or menstruation.

Chapter 5 : Five To Go: Yoga Poses Guaranteed To Increase Your Energy

You might think that yoga is all about being relaxing and soothing. But yoga poses, like the ones below, are actually energizing as well. The poses encourage your heart to get pumping and raise your energy levels as a result.

General tips:

You can do these energizing yoga poses in a super set.

It is important to pay attention to your breathing as you transition from one pose to another.

To get more energizing benefits out of the poses, you might consider performing each of them twice in a row.

Don't push yourself too far. The goal is to increase your energy, not to tire yourself out.

Yoga poses for increased energy:

COBRA POSE

Benefits:

This yoga pose strengthens your neck, chest, shoulders, and upper back.

The cobra pose also has the ability to stretch your spine, which improves your mid-back as well as upper back's mobility.

Steps:

1. Lie down on your stomach, keeping your hands on the yoga mat by your chest area.

2. Press the tops of your feet into the mat with your toes pointing backwards. Make sure to keep your legs close to each other.

3. Bend your elbows in by your sides while you gradually raise your chest and head off the mat. Do not lift your pelvis off of the floor; keep your chin slightly tucked.

4. Gaze forward and hold for one minute.

5. Breathe in while extending your body on the left and right sides before breathing out as your press down your tailbone.

6. Keep your sternum forward and up.

7. Draw your shoulder blades down your back.

Remember:

When performing this pose, see to it that your hands are rooted to the yoga mat.

BOW POSE

Benefits:

The bow pose lengthens the front part of your body while strengthening your back.

Steps:

1. Lie down on your stomach, keeping both of your arms by your sides with your palms facing up.

2. Bring your heels near your backside as you bend at the knees.

3. Extend your body as you use your hands to reach back and take hold of your ankles. Breathe out as you release your ankles.

4. Keeping your knees at a shoulder-width distance from each other, raise your heels in the opposite direction of your buttocks as you raise your thighs in the opposite direction of the mat. This position will raise both your head and upper torso off the mat.

5. Push the blades of your shoulders down and in.

6. Maintain this pose for twenty seconds to half a minute.

Remember:

Hold your gaze in front of you as you perform this pose.

Keep your chin slightly tucked in order to protect your neck.

TREE POSE

Benefits:

This balancing pose, which requires good concentration, helps strengthen your lower body muscles, especially around the knees.

Steps:

1. Begin by standing on the yoga mat with both of your hands placed on your hips.

2. Bend at the knee on your right side and then put your right foot into the nook created by your left thigh, pressing the foot against your thigh.

3. Put your hands in prayer position at your heart and hold that position for thirty seconds to one minute (or 5-7 breaths).

4. Do the same with the opposite leg.

Remember:

When performing the tree pose, make sure to hold your gaze in front of you.

CAMEL POSE

Benefits:

The camel pose allows your shoulders to become strengthened; it also increases your spine mobility.

Steps:

1. Get down on your left and right knees before placing both of your hands on your buttocks.

2. Lightly push your hips in front of you as you keep lifting your chest while carefully leaning backwards.

Remember:

Avoid leaning back too far, especially as a beginner.

Try keeping your chin close to your chest.

Be mindful of your neck and lower back when performing this pose.

SCALE POSE

Benefits:

The scale pose has the ability to effectively strengthen your hands, wrists, and abdominal muscles.

Steps:

1. Sit down on the yoga mat in a cross-legged manner.

2. Put your palms face down on the mat before lifting your torso and legs off the mat. Use your hands for balance.

Remember:

Make sure to keep your fingers spread wide to avoid straining your wrists or palms.

You can place a sturdy block between your knees for further strengthening.

Conclusion

Thank you again for downloading this book!

I hope this book was able to help you realize that yoga does not *only* help you become more relaxed and calm. Yoga is also a form of exercise that effectively helps to better your physique, place you in a more positive and self-assured mindset, move with vigor, and live a healthier life in general.

The next step is to remember that whether you are taking up yoga for reducing stress, losing weight, increasing your energy, or improving your health, it is important that you consult your doctor prior to starting any kind of routine.

I also *strongly* recommend working with a professional yoga instructor or trainer to assist you in better performing the yoga poses outlined in this guide.

Most yoga poses can be personally tailored for your body. If you do not feel good about doing a particular pose, even if it is recommended by a yoga instructor, then do not do it. And to stay on the safe side, avoid doing anything that hurts, especially if you have a problem with joint, back, or neck pain or if you have flexibility issues.

Finally, if you enjoyed this book, then I'd like to ask you for a favor. Would you be kind enough to leave a review for this book on Amazon? It would be greatly appreciated!

Thank you, and best of luck on your yoga journey!

All the best,

Catherine Walker

www.ingramcontent.com/pod-product-compliance
Lightning Source LLC
Chambersburg PA
CBHW061937280526
45787CB00004B/1635